Top 25

Nutritional

Health Supplements

Rory M. Celmin

Editor: *Ginny Greene*
Cover Design: *Rory M. Celmin*

Contact info:
email: RMCBooks@yahoo.com
twitter: @VitalityHealth9

ISBN-13: 978-0-9840186-4-2
ISBN-10: 0984018646

Legal Disclaimer: This book is intended for informational purposes only, is not meant to replace the advice or consultation of a doctor or physician and should not be construed as personal medical advice. Neither the author nor publisher is advocating, offering or participating in any health treatment, professional advice or services to the reader, nor will they be responsible for any adverse effects, damage, injury, loss or consequences allegedly arising from any information, suggestions or recommendations in this book. Readers who fail to consult appropriate health professionals assume the risk of any injuries, and should always consult their doctor or health professional for any matters relating to their health and wellbeing.

~ Table of Contents ~

Introduction...4

1. Acidophilus..6

2. Aloe Vera Juice 7

3. Apple Cider Vinegar 8

4. Bentonite...9

5. Brewer's Yeast 10

6. Calcium (chelated) 11

7. Chia Seeds.. 12

8. Coconut Oil...................................... 13

9. CoQ10... 14

10. Echinacea 15

11. Fish Oil 16

12. Garlic.. 17

13. Gingko Biloba................................ 18

14. Ginseng... 19

15. Glucosamine w/Chondroitin 20

16. Grape Seed Extract 21

17. Lecithin 22

18. Milk Thistle 23

19. Royal Jelly 24

20. Saw Palmetto.................................. 25

21. Spirulina 26

22. St. John's Wort 27

23. Turmeric 28

24. Wheatgrass Juice............................ 29

25. Whey 30

List of References..............................31-32

Resourceful Websites 33-34

Glossary..35-45

~ <u>Introduction</u> ~

Balanced nutrition is the key to optimizing health, and is done by consuming foods from a wide variety of sources. It allows us to function at our fullest potential and is often the link between diet and cancer prevention. Being proactive about staying healthy includes eating low-fat, high-fiber, nutrient-dense foods, drinking plenty of water, getting proper sleep, and about 30 minutes of cardiovascular exercise each day. Minerals are one of the basic foundations of health, but over-farming and unsustainable farming practices have left soils depleted and many people in our society mineral deficient. Nutritional deficiencies are believed to be the root of many degenerative health disorders, and may be prevented or corrected by proper nutrition because the body is a self-healing organism.

Food is the ideal source for nutrition because it is the easiest way for our body's to absorb vital nutrients. Sometimes, however, it may be beneficial to supplement nutrition. The first thing to do is determine what the purpose is for taking a nutritional supplement. Is your regular diet lacking certain nutrients that you are in need of? Are you looking for improved athletic performance or an energy boost? Taking a high-quality multivitamin is a great place to start, ensuring the basic requirements of nutrition are being met. Paying attention to what you eat and learning how your body benefits or reacts to certain foods or supplements is crucial in knowing how nutrition relates specifically to you. Preventative health should be a dietary priority for everyone, and may be the solution for many common health disorders.

Today, the American diet consists of more canned, processed, microwaveable and fast foods which are far less nutritious but have become commonplace. These foods are usually higher in sodium, sugar, white flour, saturated fats and hydrogenated vegetable oils which are all linked to an increased risk of many health disorders. Additionally, the modern-day domestication of farm animals has led to injections of growth hormones, much higher levels of saturated fat and scarce amounts of omega 3's compared to their free-range counterparts of the past.

In the United States, over a billion pounds of poisonous herbicides and pesticides are sprayed on our food crops every year. Even though they are somewhat effective for their intended purpose, most of these powerful chemicals are absorbed into the air, soil and our water supply which eventually leaches into our food supply. Organic farming increases the nutritional content of food, improves soil quality, and will help slow the toxic trend of chemical additives. It increases crop tolerance to drought, and protects the ecosystem by encouraging diverse plant and wildlife. Organic certification is the public's assurance that products have been grown in accordance with national organic standards, and helps maintain organic integrity. Obtaining proper nutrition from locally grown food is ideal, however supplementing nutrition has shown to be an effective way to further improve health and increase longevity. The following 25 nutritional supplements are the listed alphabetically, and are considered the most important health supplements available today.

1. Acidophilus – (Lactobacillus acidophilus) Acidophilus is a healthful bacterium most commonly found in the small intestines that help normalize digestion and maintain intestinal flora. Also known as *probiotics,* these 'friendly bacteria' cultures are known to promote gastrointestinal health, improve liver function, alleviate the effects of allergies, and assist in the production of vitamin K. Since 70% of the cells of our immune system are found in the digestive tract, it is important to maintain proper digestive health for a strong immune system. Acidophilus has been used to improve a myriad of digestive disorders including colitis, diarrhea, flatulence and ulcers, to protect against urinary tract and yeast infections, and may even reduce the risk of colon cancer. It is an effective and widely-used nutritional supplement that is available in capsule, tablet, liquid or powder form, and also found in foods such as yogurt and kefir. Yogurt is an ideal food source rich in acidophilus, and has been consumed throughout the Middle East since the 13th century. It is loaded with vitamins and minerals, and has been effective for lowering blood pressure and LDL (bad) cholesterol levels while increasing HDL (good) cholesterol. Yogurt is one of the smartest digestive health food choices available...and topped with berries or fruit, provides a delicious, nutritious dessert substitute for ice cream.

2. Aloe Vera Juice – (vitamins A, B1, B2, B6, B12, C & E, calcium, magnesium & zinc) For thousands of years, the aloe vera plant has been used topically to improve skin conditions, as a remedy for sunburns and as a natural moisturizer. It has also been used to alleviate acne, blemishes, burns, cuts, insect stings, infections, skin cancer and other dermatologic disorders. Unknown to most people, pure aloe vera juice is a remarkable health supplement that is consumed as a beverage and provides countless health benefits. It's sugar free, and contains numerous phytonutrients and amino acids necessary for optimal health and longevity. Aloe vera juice is alkaline, which helps restore the body back to proper pH levels. It is beneficial for improving lung function, and has shown promise in protecting against not only lung cancer, but many other forms of cancer as well. Aloe vera juice is effective for lowering cholesterol levels, alleviating arthritis and inflammation, controlling blood sugar and increasing energy. This natural remedy contains antibacterial, antifungal and antiviral properties, and increases white blood cell count which strengthens the immune system. Many studies have shown that aloe vera juice helps slow the progression of the AIDS virus by increasing T-4 cell count and lowering P-24 antigen activity. Additionally, aloe vera juice is beneficial for digestive disorders such as colitis, heartburn, IBS, indigestion, hemorrhoids and ulcers, promotes cell regeneration, detoxifies the organs and bloodstream, and increases circulation in the extremities.

3. Apple Cider Vinegar – (vitamins A, B1, B2, C & E, calcium, magnesium, potassium, sulfur, zinc) Utilized by the ancient Egyptians around 3000 BC, apple cider vinegar is a powerful detoxifying supplement that is beneficial for improving a long list of health disorders. High-quality vinegar will be organic, unfiltered with a brownish hue and contain many beneficial nutrients. Apple cider vinegar is one of the richest sources of amino acids known, and helpful for alleviating allergies, improving memory and protecting the mind from various forms of dementia such as senility and Alzheimer's disease. It is also beneficial for normalizing digestive disorders like constipation and irritable bowel syndrome, improving skin disorders such as eczema and psoriasis, and easing migraine headaches. Apple cider vinegar helps reduce the effects of food poisoning, improves bacterial, fungal, viral and yeast infections, and is powerful against pneumonia. It has also been effective for alleviating arthritis and inflammation, lowering blood pressure and cholesterol, and stimulating weight loss by breaking down fats. Even though apple cider vinegar is acidic before ingested, it has an alkaline food ash after digestion and helps reduce acidity in the body.

4. Bentonite (*montmorillonite*) – (calcite, feldspar, gypsum, magnesium)

Bentonite is a natural clay mineral sourced from the residue of weathered volcanic ash, and contains over 70 trace minerals beneficial for increasing the absorption of nutrients and improving a variety of health disorders. Ancient civilizations like the Indians of the high Andes, the aborigines of Australia and various tribes in Africa have used Bentonite clay to improve intestinal disorders and detoxify the body. It is able to absorb free radicals like a sponge which makes it one of the most effective, naturally detoxifying substances available. Bentonite's ability to bind and neutralize toxins has an electrical aspect to it; minerals are negatively charged while toxins are positively charged, so the clay's attraction is magnetic and draws toxins to it. The clay contains fine molecules that have a greater surface area, which gives it stronger absorbing or pulling power. Bentonite is an effective colon and liver cleanser, may help reduce the risk of cirrhosis and hepatitis, and helps the body recover from radiation therapy. It is also beneficial for improving digestive disorders such as constipation, diarrhea and irritable bowel syndrome, and eliminating intestinal parasites. Bentonite is available in capsule, liquid or powder form, and is most effective when consumed on an empty stomach or a couple hours after meals. When taken with psyllium (husk of psyllium seed which acts as a bulking agent), the pair create an effective natural option for detoxifying the body, digestive cleansing, maintaining regularity and lowering cholesterol levels.

5. <u>Brewer's Yeast</u> – (<u>vitamins B1, B2, B3, B6, B9, B12, chromium, copper, selenium, zinc</u>) Brewer's yeast is collected as a by-product of the beer brewing process, yet is well known to have a wide range of health benefits. It is loaded with 16 amino acids, B vitamins, minerals and protein, and is low in calories, carbohydrates, fat and sodium. Brewer's yeast is also a rich source of chromium; an essential trace mineral the body needs in order to regulate blood sugar levels. It has been known to help improve a variety of disorders such as anemia, eczema, fatigue, as well as alleviating constipation, lowering cholesterol and reducing stress. Brewer's yeast has been used during radiation therapy because it enhances the immune system, and is also beneficial for improving mental clarity and efficiency. It is usually taken with water or juice, and provides a natural energy boost when taken between meals. Brewer's yeast can be added to foods like pasta, stews, rice dishes, potatoes and meats, but should be added towards the end because the cooking process may destroy its nutritional content. It can also be taken as a capsule, tablet, or as a liquid supplement. *Diabetics should consult their doctor before consuming brewer's yeast.*

6. Calcium (chelated) – Calcium is the single most abundant and important mineral in the human body, but is the most difficult for the body to absorb. As we get older our bodies absorb less calcium when it is needed the most. When the body lacks calcium, it is leached directly from the bones which may lead to osteoporosis and a number of other physiological disorders. Obtaining calcium from food sources like broccoli, cheese, milk, spinach and yogurt is always ideal, but adding a high-quality calcium supplement to the diet can be a tremendous health advantage. Chelation is a process of binding molecules together to increase nutrient absorption, which is why *chelated* calcium is such an asset to preventative health. Calcium is important for strong bones and healthy skin, proper muscle growth, normalizing heart rhythm, the transmission of nerve impulses and many other important roles on the cellular level. It is also effective for alleviating arthritis, tendon and muscle pain, stimulating weight loss and promoting proper blood clotting. Calcium citrate is a form of chelated calcium and is absorbed more quickly than calcium carbonate. However, calcium carbonate usually contains more elemental calcium than calcium citrate so it is important to read nutritional labels. Spreading out calcium intake helps increase absorption, and taking calcium before bed further increases assimilation and induces sleep. Nutrients that improve calcium absorption include essential fatty acids, vitamins A, C, D & E, boron, magnesium, manganese & phosphorus. Iron supplements inhibit calcium absorption, and should be taken separately.

7. <u>Chia Seeds</u> – (<u>vitamins A, B complex, C, D, E & K, boron,</u> <u>calcium, copper, iron, potassium, zinc</u>) Before 3000 BC, chia seeds were a staple food of the Mayans, Aztecs and Native American tribes, and were used for their amazing ability to increase energy and endurance. Known as the 'running food', they provide more nutrients for fewer calories than almost any other food and are gluten-free. Loaded with omega-3 fatty acids, chia seeds contain more protein than salmon, and help to alleviate arthritis & inflammation, improve brain function and promote muscle growth. They are an excellent source of vitamins, minerals and phytonutrients that provide extensive cardiovascular benefits. Chia seeds provide soluble and insoluble fiber that help improve digestive regularity, lower blood pressure and cholesterol levels, and support liver, breast and prostate health. They also help control blood sugar levels by slowing down how fast our bodies convert carbohydrates into sugar, and may be beneficial for those who have Type 2 diabetes. Many use chia seeds for weight loss, as they seem to help reduce food cravings and create the feeling of being full. When mixed with water or ingested, they expand and form a bulky 'chia gel' around the outside of the seed, absorbing up to 10 times their weight in water. Chia seeds are especially beneficial for athletes because they keep them well hydrated, increase endurance and help balance electrolytes. They have a nutty flavor and can be enjoyed with cereal, yogurt, on salads or baked in breads. Chia seeds are also available as a liquid capsule or in powder form.

8. Coconut Oil – (vitamins A, B2, B3, B6, B12, E & K, iron) Native to the Caribbean, Hawaii, India, Malaysia, Polynesia, Asia, the South Pacific islands, South America and Florida, coconuts are packed full of life-extending nutrients. They were once so valuable to their cultivators that they were actually traded as currency in the 16th century. The fruit of the coconut is consumed as food, milk, oil, sugar and water, and has long been a nutritional staple of these tropical civilizations. Coconut oil is made up of 90% saturated fats, but they are medium chain triglycerides so they assimilate better. It contains fewer calories than other oils so it converts into energy easier and does not accumulate in the arteries. Many nutritional benefits have been linked to the antioxidants and *lauric acid* in virgin coconut oil, such as helping to normalize blood pressure and cholesterol, improving kidney disorders, preventing premature aging and increasing bone strength. The antibacterial, antifungal and antiviral properties of coconut oil also helps protect against herpes, influenza, and may help reduce the viral susceptibility to HIV. Additional benefits include strengthening the immune system, easing digestive disorders such as IBS and indigestion, stimulating weight loss, increasing energy, reducing stress, and improving skin, hair and dental health. Coconut oil is most commonly consumed as a liquid, but is also available as a powder or softgel capsule. Mahalo!

9. CoQ10 – (coenzyme Q10) CoQ10 is one of the most effective antioxidants available that helps protect the heart, strengthen the immune system, reduce free radical damage to the cells and promote longevity. It's found in its greatest concentration in the heart, and is what helps us look and stay young and provides much needed energy for the body. The amount of CoQ10 in our bodies exists in high levels when we are born, and is at its peak when we are in our mid-twenties. However these amounts decline with age, so it is important to try and maintain appropriate levels. CoQ10 is one of the main nutrients our bodies need to produce physical energy; it transports the protons and electrons needed to produce ATP – our body's energy source. In addition to improving cardiovascular health, CoQ10 is beneficial for lowering blood pressure and cholesterol levels, may help reduce the risk of cancer and Parkinson's disease, as shows promise in protecting against senility and Alzheimer's disease. It has also been helpful for improving impotence, infertility, nausea, easing headaches and reducing the frequency of migraine headaches. CoQ10 is available as a softgel capsule, tablet, liquid or powder.

10. <u>Echinacea</u> – (<u>vitamins B1, B2, B3 & C, calcium, magnesium, phosphorus, potassium, selenium, zinc</u>) One of the most effective and respected herbal supplements today, echinacea has been used for hundreds of years to help alleviate the common cold, coughing, sore throats, fevers and the flu. Echinacea is most widely revered for its ability to stimulate the immune system by effectively strengthening white blood cells, and protecting against bacterial and viral infections. It helps minimize congestion and swelling in the lymphatic system, and works well when combined with the herb *astralagus* to stimulate immune cells. Echinacea has been used to protect against meningitis, urinary tract and yeast infections, to detoxify both circulatory and respiratory systems, and contains powerful antioxidants that help slow the aging process. It provides antibiotic benefits when applied topically, and has been effective for reducing infections and repairing wounds, and improving skin disorders such as acne, boils, eczema and psoriasis. Echinacea is available in capsule, tablet, tincture or powder form, and is also known to help alleviate inflammation. *Those who are allergic to ragweed should avoid echinacea.*

11. **Fish Oil** – (vitamin B6, folate, magnesium, phosphorus)

Fish oil supplements contain both omega-3 essential fatty acids DHA and EPA which strengthens cardiovascular health, alleviates arthritis and inflammation and lowers blood pressure and cholesterol levels. It contains powerful anti-aging properties that promote longevity, improve skin disorders and promote eye health. Fish oil has been used as a potent anti-cancer supplement beneficial for inhibiting the growth of tumors. It also helps control blood sugar levels, reduces anxiety and depression, and is associated with lower levels of senility and Alzheimer's disease. Quality food sources of omega 3 fish oil include albacore tuna, herring, mackerel, sardines, swordfish and trout. Due to its higher content of omega 3's, fish oil provides similar yet more compelling nutritional benefits than the alpha-linolenic acid (ALA) found in flaxseed oil. Cod liver oil also contains omega-3 fatty acids plus significant levels of vitamins A and D which help protect against breast, colon and prostate cancer. However, exceeding the recommended daily allowance (RDA) of vitamin A may become harmful and has been associated with birth defects. Fish oil may contain toxins such as mercury and polychlorinated biphenyls (PCB's), so be diligent when selecting this health supplement. Wild-caught salmon/fish has little to no mercury content, whereas farmed salmon/fish tends to have higher levels of mercury. Many fish oil products are purified through a distillation process, so read product labels to make sure you are getting a high-quality, mercury-free product. It is mainly taken in capsule form, but is also available as a tablet.

16

12. Garlic – (<u>vitamins A, B1, B2, B3, B6, C, calcium, magnesium, manganese, selenium and zinc</u>) Native to central Asia yet enjoyed throughout the world for over 6,000 years, garlic is one of the oldest and most highly regarded nutritional spices that has been used for improving a myriad of health disorders. Garlic was once so valuable that it was praised and used as currency by the ancient Egyptians. This highly flavorful bulb contains powerful, life-extending antioxidants that reduce the risk of heart attack and stroke, lower blood pressure and cholesterol levels, improve circulation and detoxify the blood. Garlic slows down the oxidation process of LDL cholesterol, and helps prevent saturated fats from clogging the arteries. It contains a sulfur compound called *allicin* which has been effective for destroying cancer cells, inhibiting the growth of tumors, controlling blood sugar and supporting healthy liver function. The sulfur compounds in garlic are chelators of toxins and heavy metals – attaching to them and removing them from our bodies. Furthermore, it contains antibacterial and antiviral properties, helps alleviate arthritis, asthma and bronchitis, strengthens the immune system and protects against colds, fevers and the flu. Garlic is most effective when consumed as food, but is available as a nutritional supplement in liquid capsule, powder, tablet or tincture form.

13. <u>**Ginkgo Biloba**</u> – (<u>vitamins A, B1, B2, B3 & C, calcium,</u> <u>magnesium, phosphorus, potassium, zinc</u>) Dating back to the Jurassic era and once thought to be extinct, ginkgo biloba is a rare type of tree native to China that for centuries has been utilized for its various health benefits. It is most widely known and revered for improving the effects of senility, increasing memory and promoting proper brain function. Ginkgo biloba helps reduce muscle cramps from clogged arteries, and protects against impotence by increasing circulation and tissue oxygenation. It contains powerful antioxidant properties that are beneficial for easing asthma and bronchitis, alleviating headaches and migraines, and may be helpful in reducing the risk of senility and Alzheimer's disease. Ginkgo biloba is also known to protect against kidney disorders, improve conditions of eczema, increase energy and help ease depression. Other benefits include alleviating altitude sickness, reducing PMS discomforts and protecting organs against radiation damage. Ginkgo biloba is available in capsule, tablet, liquid or powder form. *Ginkgo biloba is not recommended for those who have a lack of blood-clotting ability, or before surgery.*

14. <u>Ginseng</u> – (<u>vitamins B1, B2, B3, B9 & C, calcium, iron, magnesium, phosphorus, potassium, zinc</u>) Native to Asia and Siberia, ginseng has been revered for thousands of years in Traditional Chinese Medicine for its ability to promote proper adrenal function, alleviate symptoms of PMS as well as many other disorders. It is beneficial for relieving anxiety, depression, mood swings, stress and increases mental alertness. This nutritious spice is well known for increasing testosterone levels, sperm production and reducing the risk of erectile dysfunction. Ginseng is effective for stimulating both the immune and nervous systems, inhibiting the growth of cancer cells and lowering cholesterol levels. It is rich in folate which increases the production of red blood cells, and improves digestive disorders such as diarrhea, indigestion and ulcers. Ginseng increases circulation, energy levels and athletic endurance, and is a natural appetite suppressant. It is also effective for lowering blood sugar levels, and may help reduce the risk of senility and Alzheimer's disease. Additional benefits include alleviating arthritis, inflammation, asthma and bronchitis, and relieving symptoms of the flu and common cold. Ginseng is usually consumed as a liquid capsule or tincture, but is also available in tablet or powder form.

15. Glucosamine w/ Chondroitin

Glucosamine is a naturally occurring compound found in healthy cartilage – the strong connective tissue that cushions our joints. It supports the strength, structure and function of cartilage which makes it easier to move, and allows our bones to function with minimal friction. Glucosamine is a precursor in the synthesis of proteins and lipids, and is also found in animal bones, bone marrow and the shells of shellfish.

Chondroitin is a derivative of glucosamine that strengthens connective tissues in the body and also supports joint flexibility.

When taken together, glucosamine and chondroitin strengthen and support healthy cartilage, tendons and ligaments. They promote ease of movement, help lubricate joints and actually help rejuvenate cartilage. This allows for better joint elasticity, flexibility, mobility and support. After a period of consistent use, glucosamine and chondroitin are shown to promote long-term joint health. They are available, either separate or combined, and can be taken in capsule, tablet, tincture or powder form.

16. <u>Grape Seed Extract</u> – (<u>vitamin E, flavonoids, linoleic acid, resveratrol</u>) Grape seed extract is a liquid derivative of the grape seed and is one of the most powerful antioxidants nature provides. Belonging to a class of phytonutrients called *bioflavonoids*, it is beneficial for lowering blood pressure and cholesterol, improving cardiovascular health and protecting against premature aging. Grape seed extract is especially beneficial for athletes because it binds to collagen fibers increasing muscle flexibility and strengthening the elasticity of ligaments and tendons. This nutrient-dense supplement helps protect cells from toxins caused by pollution, smoking, stress and other environmental factors. Grape seed extract increases circulation, reduces the formation of plaque in the arteries that leads to arteriosclerosis and atherosclerosis, and may be beneficial for those who suffer from senility or Alzheimer's disease because it increases mental alertness. It is also effective for alleviating arthritis and inflammation, protecting against Parkinson's disease, and reducing the risk of cancer. Furthermore, grape seed extract supports liver and kidney health, improves digestive function, promotes eye health and helps eliminate bacterial and viral infections. It is mostly consumed as a liquid tincture or softgel capsule, but is also available in tablet and powder form.

17. <u>Lecithin</u> – (<u>vitamins B1, B2 & C</u>) A brow-yellowish fatty substance naturally occurring in animal and plant tissues, egg yolks and soy beans, lecithin plays an important role in optimizing health. It stimulates weight loss by breaking down fats in the body, and helps prevent fat accumulation in the liver which protects against cirrhosis and hepatitis. Lecithin is extremely important for managing the flow of nutrients and waste materials in and out of cells. It is beneficial for lowering blood pressure and cholesterol levels, improving cardiovascular health, and reducing the risk of atherosclerosis by protecting against plaque buildup in the arteries. Along with its main component choline, lecithin is known for improving women's reproductive health, supporting a healthy pregnancy, promoting proper infant growth, sustaining healthy breast cells and easing the discomforts of menopause. It is also beneficial for men's reproductive health because it is a major component of sperm, and soy lecithin supplements have been found to increase the volume of prostate secretions. Furthermore, lecithin has been used for fibromyalgia and multiple sclerosis (MS), to protect against gallstones and pancreatitis, to help alleviate narcolepsy and improve conditions of psoriasis. Last but not least, it is effective for improving brain function and may help reduce the risk of dementia. Lecithin is available in capsule, tablet, liquid or powder form.

18. **Milk Thistle** – (calcium, iron, magnesium, manganese, phosphorus, potassium, selenium, zinc) The liver is the 2nd largest organ, and acts as a filter for cleaning toxins out of our bodies. Milk thistle is known to help improve a variety of degenerative disorders, but is especially known for its positive effects on the liver. It contains powerful antioxidants that help normalize enzyme levels, and protects the liver and kidneys from damage caused by alcohol, environmental toxins, viruses and over-the-counter pain relievers (acetaminophen, ibuprofen etc.) Milk thistle contains *silymarin*, a natural substance known to help regenerate damaged liver cells and tissues, and is important for those with cirrhosis or hepatitis. It is beneficial for strengthening the immune system, reducing the risk of atherosclerosis, and protecting against bladder, breast, colon, lung and prostate cancer. Milk thistle has also been effective for normalizing metabolism, improving adrenal, digestive and gallbladder function, increasing the absorption of nutrients and maintaining healthy blood quality. It enables the liver to process estrogen more effectively which helps women who suffer from infertility. Many athletes and bodybuilders who use performance-enhancing supplements (anabolic steroids, prohormones, thermogenics) take milk thistle to reduce stress on the liver. Milk thistle is usually consumed in capsule, tincture or powder form, but is also available as a tablet.

19. Royal Jelly – (vitamins B5, B6 & C, zinc) Royal jelly is a milky substance secreted from young worker bees between their 6th and 12th days of life. When these special nurse bees combine honey and pollen, they naturally create royal jelly. Rich in DNA, RNA, enzymes, hormones, protein, vitamins and minerals, royal jelly acts as a catalyst for cell regeneration, contains powerful anti-tumor properties and strengthens the immune system. It is a rich source of collagen and zinc which protects against osteoporosis by enhancing the formation of bone tissue, and contains the compound (10H2DA) that has shown to inhibit joint destruction beneficial for those who suffer from arthritis, inflammation and gout. Royal jelly increases red blood cell count, improves blood quality beneficial for those who are anemic, and protects against atherosclerosis by helping to prevent the narrowing of the arteries. It is effective for lowering cholesterol, and is a great source of glucose and fructose, and helps stabilize blood-sugar levels. Loaded with amino acids and various phytonutrients, royal jelly is beneficial for autoimmune disorders such as lupus, fibromyalgia, multiple sclerosis (MS) and Parkinson's disease. It also helps protect against cirrhosis and hepatitis, enhances sexual vitality, increases energy, and is one of the most effective carbohydrates to take before exercise. Royal jelly is known as 'brain food', and has been used for easing anxiety, depression and migraine headaches, as well as protecting against senility and Alzheimer's disease. Possessing antibacterial, antifungal and antiviral properties, it also improves skin disorders like acne, eczema and canker sores. Royal jelly comes in capsule, tablet, liquid or powder form.

20. <u>Saw Palmetto</u> – (beta carotene, fatty acids, tannins) Saw palmetto is a small palm-type shrub native to the Atlantic and Gulf coastal plains, and is also grown in southern Europe and Africa as well. The dark purple-colored fruit from this tree was used by Native Americans to improve a variety of digestive and genital disorders. Increasingly popular in Europe, saw palmetto is used as an antiseptic, diuretic, expectorant, sedative, for easing menstrual discomforts and as a tonic for soothing the digestive tract. This herbal extract is known to lower the risk of prostate cancer by its ability to shrink the prostate gland and inhibit cancerous cell growth within the inner lining of the prostate. Saw palmetto helps suppress the production of *dihydrotestosterone* (DHT), a form of testosterone the body produces that causes enlargement of the prostate gland. It contains fatty acids that help alleviate symptoms of testicular and urinary inflammation, support healthy hormone levels, protect against impotence and infertility, increase sexual stamina and may be beneficial for improving male pattern baldness. Saw palmetto can be taken as a capsule, tablet, liquid or in powder form.

21. Spirulina – (<u>vitamins B1, B2, B3, C & E, calcium, chromium, magnesium, potassium, selenium, zinc</u>) Thriving in hot climates around the world, spirulina is a microalgae consisting of vegetable proteins, chlorophyll, dietary fiber and many other healthful nutrients. It contains more beta carotene than carrots, a higher concentration of protein than soybeans, and contains a rare fatty acid called *gamma-linolenic acid* (GLA). Spirulina is found in mother's milk and is essential for the proper development of healthy babies. It is rich in amino acids, B vitamins, various minerals and other essential nutrients that help reduce the risk of cancer, lower blood pressure and cholesterol, and strengthen the immune system. An excellent source of natural energy, spirulina promotes healthy nerves and tissues, increases nutrient absorption and detoxifies the kidneys. It also protects against anemia, and is beneficial for those who are diabetic or hypoglycemic because it helps stabilize blood sugar when taken between meals. Spirulina is available as a capsule, tablet, liquid or powder.

22. <u>St. John's Wort</u> – (<u>vitamin C, fatty acids, tannins</u>) Native to Asia, Europe and North America, St. John's Wort was utilized for thousands of years for improving a variety of topical disorders such as bruising, burns, dermatitis, skin cancer, snake bites and wounds. It is most commonly used as an anti-depressant and to reduce stress, but is also effective for relieving urinary tract infections, diarrhea and improving jaundice. St. John's Wort helps support the immune system, and contains antiviral properties which may be beneficial for those with HIV & AIDS. Rich in phytonutrients, St. John's Wort has been used to protect bone marrow from radiation damage, to reduce swelling of the tendons, and help relieve pain associated with carpal tunnel syndrome (CTS). Excellent when seeped as a tea, it is effective against tooth decay, and contains antibiotic properties that help alleviate bronchitis, congestion, phlegm, sinus infections and peptic ulcers. As a nutritional supplement, St. John's Wort is available in capsule or tincture form, but is also available as a powder or tablet.

23. Turmeric – (vitamins B1, B2, B3 & C, calcium, potassium, zinc)
Originating in western India and utilized as flavoring, as a dye, and as medicine since 600 BC, turmeric is a powerful antioxidant that has been used to reduce the risk of leukemia, as well as colon, breast, lung, ovarian, pancreatic, prostate, stomach and skin cancer. Its active ingredient, *curcumin,* is beneficial for lowering cholesterol, alleviating arthritis, inflammation, asthma, bronchitis, relieving cystic fibrosis, and helps strengthen the cardiovascular system. Most commonly found in yellow curry and mustards, turmeric improves liver health, strengthens the immune system and helps relieve the effects of food poisoning. This powerful super-spice helps increase blood circulation, improve intestinal flora, eliminate intestinal parasites and reduce the risk of developing polyps in the colon. Turmeric has shown promise in breaking up the beta-amyloid plaques collected in the brain, which is considered one of the main causes of Alzheimer's disease. The elderly people of India rarely develop dementia or Alzheimer's, which is believed to be related to their regular consumption of turmeric. It is available in capsule, tablet, tincture and powder form, and is also seeped as tea.

24. <u>Wheatgrass Juice</u> – (<u>vitamins A, C & E, calcium, iron, magnesium, phosphorus, potassium, protein</u>) Wheatgrass juice is considered the nectar of life, and is one of the most healthful nutritional supplements available! Green drinks are rich in vitamins, minerals, enzymes, antioxidants, provide phytonutrients to every cell in the body, protect our DNA and contain powerful anti-aging properties. Chlorophyll is the green pigment found in plants, is the first product of light and contains more light energy than any other element. Wheatgrass juice is about 70% chlorophyll and is an excellent blood cleanser. The molecular structure of chlorophyll resembles that of the oxygen-carrying protein hemoglobin and is considerably adaptable to our blood. The human body functions best when it is highly oxygenated - wheatgrass juice increases the amount of oxygen in the bloodstream promoting cardiovascular health. It improves conditions of anemia, helps control blood sugar levels, and detoxifies the kidneys and liver. Wheatgrass juice is effective for lowering blood pressure and cholesterol, protecting against most forms of cancer, and provides a natural energy boost. It helps restore vitality by removing heavy metals like lead, mercury and arsenic from the body, and is believed to help slow the process of graying hair. Additional benefits include alleviating arthritis and inflammation, reducing inner ear infections, improving acne, eczema and psoriasis, cleaning the lymph system and protecting against tooth decay. Wheatgrass juice is easily absorbed and most effective when supplemented as a liquid, but is also available in capsule, tablet and powder form. It's time to go green!

25. <u>Whey Protein</u> – (<u>amino acids</u>) Whey is the liquid that remains after milk has been curdled and strained, and contains the highest quality protein that nature provides. Since protein builds muscle, whey protein is one of the most popular nutritional supplements among athletes and bodybuilders because it contains all the essential amino acids your body needs for muscle growth. It is beneficial when consumed before training because whey protein absorbs into the bloodstream much quicker than most other types of protein. Whey protein is also ideal for post-workout nutrition because it keeps amino acids levels elevated, and muscles need plenty of high-quality protein to continue to build, repair and maintain muscle mass. It is usually supplemented as a powder or tincture, but is also available in capsules or as tablets.

(Creatine is another popular protein supplement. It is a specific amino acid that our bodies convert into creatine phosphate for storage in the muscles. During short periods of high-intensity exercise, creatine phosphate is then converted to ATP - one of the bodies most important and efficient energy sources. However, creatine tends to fill muscles with water, and post-workout may decrease muscle rigidity)

~ List of References ~

*Anderson, Jean E. M.S., Deskins, Barbara Ph.D. *The Nutrition Bible – A Comprehensive No-Nonsense Guide to Foods, Nutrients, Additives, Preservatives, Pollutants and Everything Else We Eat and Drink.* New York, NY: HarperCollins Publishers, 1997

*Balch, Phyllis A., CNC. *Prescription for Nutritional Healing, 5th edition.* New York, NY: Penguin Group (Avery), 2010

*Beck, Leslie R.D. *Leslie Beck's Nutrition Encyclopedia.* Toronto, Ontario: Penguin Group, 2003

*Campbell, T. Colin, Ph.D., and Campbell, Thomas M. *The China Study – Startling Implications for Diet, Weight Loss and Long-term Health.* Dallas, TX: BenBella Books, 2005

*Chmelik, Stefan. *Chinese Herbal Secrets – The Key to Total Health.* New York, NY: The Ivy Press Limited, 1999

*Colbert, Don M.D. *Toxic Relief – Restore Health and Energy Through Fasting and Detoxification.* Lake Mary, FL: Siloam Press, 2003

*Kirschmann, Gayla J. and Kirschmann, John D. *Nutrition Almanac, 4th edition.* New York, NY: McGraw-Hill, 1996

*Miller, David Niven. *Grow Youthful – A Practical Guide to Slowing Your Aging.* Cottesloe, West Australia: John Hunt Publishing & O-Books, 2007

*Murray, Michael N.D. and Pizzorno, Joseph N.D. with Pizzorno, Lara M.A., L.M.T. *The Encyclopedia of Healing Foods.* New York, NY: Atria Books, 2005

*Plasker, Eric D.C. *The 100 Year Lifestyle.* Avon, MA: Adams Media Publishing, 2007

*Price, Weston A., D.D.S. *Nutrition and Physical Degeneration, 8th edition.* San Diego, CA: Price-Pottenger Nutrition Foundation, 2008

*Roizen, Michael F., M.D. and Oz, Mehmet C., M.D. *You Staying Young – The Owners Manual for Extending Your Warranty.* New York, NY: Free Press, 2007

*Somer, Elizabeth M.A., R.D. *Food & Mood – The Complete Guide to Eating Well and Feeling Your Best, 2nd edition.* New York, NY: Owl Books, 1999

*Tessmer, Kimberly A. R.D., L.D. *The Everything Nutrition Book – Boost Energy, Prevent Illness and Live Longer.* Avon, MA: Adams Media, 2003

*Trattler, Ross N.D., D.O. and Jones, Adrian N.D. *Better Health Through Natural Healing, 2nd edition.* Heatherton VIC, Australia: Hinkler Books, 2001

*Trowell, Hubert C. and Burkitt, Denis P. *Western Diseases: Their Emergence and Prevention.* Cambridge, MA: Harvard University Press, 1981

*Wilson, Dr. Lawrence. *Legal Guidelines for Unlicensed Practitioners.* Prescott, AZ: L.D. Wilson Consultants, 2007

*Yeager, Selene. *The Doctor's Book of Food Remedies.* Emmaus, PA: Rodale Press Inc., 2000

~ <u>Resourceful Websites</u> ~

Administration on Aging (AOA) – www.aoa.gov

Alzheimer's Association – www.alz.org

American Cancer Society (ACS) – www.cancer.org

American Diabetes Association (ADA) – www.diabetes.org

American Heart Association (AHA) – www.americanheart.org

American Institute for Cancer Research (AICR) – www.aicr.org

American Society for Nutrition (ASN) – www.nutrition.org

Cancer Cure Foundation – www.cancure.org

Center for Nutrition Policy and Promotion (CNPP) –
www.cnpp.usda.gov/dietaryguidelines.htm

Daily Green – www.thedailygreen.com

Desert Harvest – www.desertharvest.com

Everyday Health – www.everydayhealth.com

Eden Organic – www.edenfoods.com

Hippocrates Health Institute (HHI) – www.hippocratesinst.org

IDEA Health and Fitness Association – www.ideafit.com

Immune Deficiency Foundation (IDF) – www.primaryimmune.org

Institute of Food Technologists (IFT) – www.ift.org

Live Strong – www.livestrong.com

Linus Pauling Institute-Oregon State University – www.lpi.oregonstate.edu

Local Harvest – www.localharvest.org

Medical News Today – www.medicalnewstoday.com

Mayo Clinic – www.mayoclinic.com

Mental Health America (MHA) – www.nmha.org

National Academy of Sciences (NAS) – www.nationalacademies.org

National Association for Health and Fitness – www.physicalfitness.org

National Cancer Institute (NCI) – www.cancer.gov

National Center for Complementary and Alternative Medicine (NCCAM) – www.nccam.nih.gov

National Council on Aging (NCOA) – www.ncoa.org

National Institutes of Health – www.nih.gov

Natural Health Research Institute (NHRI) – www.naturalhealthresearch.org

National Kidney Foundation (NKF) – www.kidney.org

Nutrition.gov – www.nutrition.gov

National Osteoporosis Foundation (NOF) – www.nof.org

Oasis Advanced Wellness – www.oasisadvancedwellness.com

Okinawa Centenarian Study (OCS) – www.okicent.org

Organic Authority – www.organicauthority.com

The Organic Center – www.organic-center.org

Organic Consumers Association (OCA) – www.organicconsumers.org

Organic Trade Association (OTA) – www.ota.com

Traditional Chinese Medicine (TCM) – www.chinesemedicineherbs.net

United States Department of Agriculture (USDA) – www.usda.gov

University of Texas at Galveston | Medical Branch (UTMB) – www.utmb.edu

USDA National Agricultural Library – www.fnic.nal.usda.gov

WebMD – www.webmd.com

Whole Foods Market – www.wholefoodsmarket.com

~ <u>Glossary</u> ~

A

Absorption – the process of assimilating nutrients into the body

Adaptogen – herbal substances that reduce stress and produce beneficial adjustments in the body

Alpha-carotene – a phytonutrient found in carrots that is beneficial for eye health

Alpha-linolenic acid (ALA) – omega-3 essential fatty acid found in flaxseed, pumpkin & soybean oils

Amino acid – nitrogen and carbon-based organic compounds that build protein and muscle

Anabolic – substance that helps convert nutrition into building and repairing muscle tissues in the body

Antacid – a substance that neutralizes stomach acid

Antibody – immune system protein that combats bacteria, fungus and other foreign substances

Antigen – a substance that provokes the creation of antibodies

Antihistamine – a substance that binds with histamine receptors and reduces the effects of histamines

Antioxidant – a substance that minimizes free radical damage to the heart, arteries, and tissues, such as vitamins, minerals and nutrients

Arachidonic acid (AA) – an omega-6 essential fatty acid found in eggs, meat, poultry and shellfish

Ascorbic acid – the organic compound known as vitamin C

B

Beta carotene – phytonutrient with antioxidant properties the body uses to produce vitamin A, found in broccoli, carrots, collard greens, kale, pumpkin, spinach and sweet potatoes

Bio-availability – the ease of which nutrients can be absorbed into the body

Bioflavonoid – a group of active substances essential for the absorption of vitamin C

Blood sugar – concentration of glucose in the blood

C

Carbohydrate – organic substances that are our the main source of energy in our diets

Carcinogen – a toxic substance capable of producing cancer

Carotene – a substance that is converted into vitamin A in the body

Cartenoids – phytonutrients that contain antioxidant properties

Cellulose – an organic carbohydrate from fruits and vegetables

Chelation – chemical process where molecules bind to a mineral atom increasing its bio-availability

Chelation therapy – the introduction of substances into the body to remove heavy metals

Chlorophyll – the green pigment in plants that is vital for photosynthesis; converting light into energy

Cholesterol – steroid metabolite compound including lipids (fats) naturally produced by the body, a structural component of cell membranes, helps absorption of fatty acids; HDL (good) and LDL (bad)

Citric acid – organic acid found in citrus fruits

Coenzyme – a substance that works with enzymes to promote normal enzyme activity

Complete protein – a protein that contains all 8 essential amino acids

Complex carbohydrate – a carbohydrate that provides fiber and slowly releases sugar into the body

Conjugated Linoleic Acid (CLA) – a naturally occurring fatty-acid that helps reduce body fat

Cordyceps – rare medicinal mushroom used in Traditional Chinese Medicine for over 5,000 years to strengthen the immune system, improve adrenal function, lower blood pressure and cholesterol, prevent kidney disease and liver disorders

Cortisol – one of the main catabolic hormones in the body

Creatine – a high-energy compound in muscle cells which stores energy and increases strength

Cruciferous – 'cross-shaped' blossoms that support digestive health (broccoli, cabbage, cauliflower)

D

Detoxification – process of eliminating toxic substances from the body

Diuretic – substance that increases urine flow

Docosahexaenoic acid (DHA) – an omega-3 essential fatty acid found in marine micro-algae, anchovies, cod, mackerel, salmon and tuna

E

Eicosapentaenoic acid (EPA) – an omega-3 essential fatty acid found in cod, salmon, sardines and tuna

Electrolytes (potassium, sodium and chloride) – soluble substances containing free ions that are capable of conducting electric impulses throughout the body

Enzyme – a protein catalyst that manages or increases chemical reactions in the body

Essential Fatty Acids (EFA's) – amino acids that cannot be synthesized by the body and must be supplied by foods or supplements

F

Fat-soluble – the ability to dissolve in fats and oils

Fatty acid – a carboxylic acid derived from natural fats and oils

Fiber – indigestible plant matter that helps eliminate toxins from the body (fruits, vegetables, nuts, legumes, whole grains)

Flavonoid – a class of metabolite substances found in plants that help protect against cancer

Fructose – a sugar found in fruit that has a low glycemic index

G

Gamma-linolenic acid (GLA) – an omega-6 essential fatty acid found in borage & primrose oil

Gland – an organ that synthesizes substances for release into the bloodstream

Glucose – a simple sugar in the blood that is the major energy source for the body's cells and functions

Gluten – a protein found in oats, wheat, barley and rye

Glycemic Index (GI) – measure of how much food raises blood sugar levels as compared to white bread, which has a GI of 100 (the lower the number the less insulin is released by the body)

Glycogen – the main form of glucose stored in the body, then converts back to glucose to supply energy

Growth Hormone (GH) – a hormone that is released by the pituitary gland that promotes muscle growth and the breakdown of body fat for energy, subsides with age

H

HDL cholesterol (high-density lipoprotein) – known as *good cholesterol*, it helps clear fat from the bloodstream and indicates a low risk of cardiovascular disease

Heavy metals (arsenic, cadmium, lead, mercury) – elements that possess metallic properties and have a gravity measurement greater than 5.0

Herbal therapy – herbal combination of tinctures, extracts and capsules used for cleansing and healing

Histamine – chemical released by the immune system that has potential negative effects on the body

Homeopathy – alternative medicines using herbs, natural substances to strengthen the immune system

Hormone – vital substances produced by the body that regulates many biological processes

Hydrochloric acid (HCL) – a strong corrosive stomach acid that helps digestion

Hydrogenation – process by which hydrogen atoms are combined with oil molecules to turn liquid oils into solids, destroying the nutritional value of the oil

Hypoallergenic – having a low capacity for being affected by allergies

I

Immune system – a complex system of organs, cells and proteins that protect the body against disease

Inorganic – substances that do not contain carbon

Insulin – an anabolic hormone produced by the pancreas that regulates proper blood sugar levels

Intestinal flora – friendly bacteria in the digestive tract that are essential for digestion and metabolism

Isoflavones – a class of phytonutrients that protect against estrogen-based cancers like breast cancer

K

Kefir – fermented milk product that contains anti-aging properties

Ketosis – a process of metabolism where the liver converts fats into fatty acids and is used for energy

Kombucha – a sweetened fermented tea beverage that has detoxifying effects and healing properties

L

Lactase – an enzyme that converts lactose into glucose and is necessary for digesting milk and dairy

Lactic acid – an acid created from glucose metabolism that accumulates in the body after strenuous exercise causing muscle fatigue and pain

Lactose – term referring to milk sugar

Lauric acid – a fatty acid found in coconut and palm kernel oil that has antimicrobial properties

LDL cholesterol (low density lipoprotein) – known as *bad cholesterol* that may cause cardiovascular disease

Legumes – seed pod that splits both sides when ripe (alfalfa, beans, carob, lentils, peanuts, peas, soy)

Lentils – a leguminous, climbing-vine plant containing only 2 seeds to a pod (beluga, black, green, red, white, yellow)

Liminoids – phytonutrients found in citrus fruits that help inhibit the production of cancer cells and HIV protease activity

Linolenic acid (LA) – an omega-6 essential fatty acid found in corn oil, safflower and sunflower oil

Lipids – natural substances that are soluble in the same solvents as fats and oils

Lipolysis – refers to the chemical breakdown of body fat by enzymes that produce energy

Lipoprotein – protein molecule that helps transport fats around the bloodstream

Lipotropic – substances that help break down fat during metabolism and manage blood sugar levels

Lutein – phytonutrient that helps protect against macular degeneration (spinach, kale, turnip greens)

Lycopene – a phytonutrient that helps protect against prostate cancer and ultraviolet rays from the sun found in guava, pink grapefruit, tomatoes and watermelon

M

Macrobiotics – referring to a branch of Eastern medicine that uses grain as a staple food, and balances Yin (negative) and Yang (positive) foods together to overcome health issues

Macronutrients (proteins, carbohydrates and fats) – essential elements needed in large quantities to sustain proper health

Malabsorption – the inability to absorb nutrients from the intestines into the bloodstream

Metabolism – process by which cells absorb nutrition and change food into energy

Mineral – naturally occurring substance that is essential for human life and vital to metabolic processes

Monounsaturated fats (canola, olive, peanut and sunflower oils) – fatty acids that are not saturated with hydrogen, typically liquid at room temperature but will solidify when refrigerated

N

Naturopathy – alternative form of medicine using a combination of natural methods to combat disease and maintain health

Nonessential Amino Acids – amino acids that can be produced by the body from other amino acids, therefore not essential to the human diet

Nutrient – a natural substance that all living organisms need for growth and survival

Nutrition – the science of turning food into fuel for the body to use

O

Organic – referring to foods that are grown naturally, without the use of synthetic chemicals like herbicides, pesticides or hormones

Oxalates (oxalic acid) – organic substances found in humans, plants and animals of which high concentrations may lead to kidney stones; (oxalic acid foods include: amaranth, beans, beet greens, beer, berries, celery, chocolate, figs, kale, kiwi, leeks, nuts/seeds, okra, parsley, plums, quinoa, rhubarb, soy foods, spinach, squash, Swiss chard, tangerines, watercress, wheat germ)

P

Parasite – a smaller organism living on/inside of a larger host, it is completely dependent on its host for nourishment and can be potentially damaging

Pepsin – a digestive enzyme released by the stomach to break down food proteins into peptides

Peptide – a compound made up of two or more amino acids that are broken down by protein molecules

pH (potential of hydrogen) – a measurement of the acidity and alkalinity of a substance or solution

Photosynthesis – the synthesis of organic compounds from inorganic compounds by plants and algae involving light energy

Phytonutrients – natural substances found in fruits and vegetables that protect the body against disease (chlorophyll, carotenoids, flavonoids, isoflavones, inositol, lignans, indoles, phenols, sulfides, terpenes)

Polyphenols – a group of compounds found in plants that have at least one phenol unit per molecule

Polysaccharides – a class of carbohydrates which breaks down during hydrolysis to a monosaccharide

Probiotics – substances that promote the growth of friendly bacteria in the body

Protein – nitrogen-based organic compounds made from amino acids that are the basic components of animal and vegetable tissues, needed for growth and repair

Proteolytic enzymes – enzymes that break down proteins and reduce the risk of cancer

Purines – natural substances that are part of the chemical structure of human, plant and animal genes, high concentrations may lead to arthritis, gout and inflammation (purine-rich foods include: anchovies, asparagus, bacon, beef, cauliflower, chicken, eggs, ham, herring, mackerel, mushrooms, mussels, oatmeal, organ meats, peas, pork, sardines, shellfish, smelt, spinach, sweetbreads, turkey, yeast),

R

RDA (Recommended Daily Allowance) – the basic amount of nutrients that should be consumed daily to maintain proper health

Retinoic acid – the acid from vitamin A

S

Saliva – a mixture of water, protein and salts that makes food easy to swallow and digest

Saturated fat (butter, chocolate, dairy, lard, meat) – regarded as unhealthy fat, it is typically solid at room temperature and has been shown to raise cholesterol levels

Simple carbohydrate – a carbohydrate that is quickly digested and absorbed into the bloodstream

Stevia – a natural herbal sweetener native to South America that is much sweeter that sugar

Sucrose – table sugar

Synergy – the harmonious interaction between two or more substances where their combined ability is greater than their individual actions

T

Thermogenics – dietary supplements that increase metabolism and generate heat

Thyroid gland – internal thermostat regulating body temperature by secreting hormones that control energy used and calories burned

Tolerance – the capability of an organism to endure an unfavorable environment

Toxin – a poison that impairs health and bodily functions

Trace element – mineral required by the body in minute quantities for proper growth and development

Trans-fat – unsaturated fat produced through hydrogenation; increases risk of cardiovascular disease

Triglyceride – compound made up of three fatty acids and glycerol and is how fat is stored in the body

U

Unsaturated fat (olive, flaxseed, safflower and fish oils) – known as healthy fat, these help reduce cholesterol and triglycerides levels in the blood

V

Vitamin – organic substance obtained through diet to maintain proper health and support many biological functions

W

Water-soluble – the ability to dissolve in water

X

Xylitol – a natural sweetener made from birch bark that has antifungal properties, has a low glycemic index (GI) score and alkalizes the body

Y

Yang (heat, light and dryness) – one of two essential principles of Chinese medicine needed to create balance and harmony in the body, organs include the gallbladder, spleen, intestines and skin

Yin (cold, shadow and moisture) – the other essential principle of Chinese medicine needed to create balance and harmony in the body, organs include the liver, heart, kidneys, lungs and bones

Z

Zeaxanthin – a phytonutrient that protects against macular degeneration found in citrus fruits, eggs and green vegetables

~ __About the Author__ ~

Rory M. Celmin is certified in sports nutrition from the International Fitness Professional Association (IFPA), received a Bachelor's Degree in English from California State University San Marcos (CSUSM) and has studied health and nutrition for over 20 years. He is the founder of Vitality Health Solutions, authored *Nature's Nutrition – A Comprehensive Resource Guide for Super Foods, Natural Supplements and Preventative Health*, and in his spare time he enjoys surfing, basketball, tennis, hiking and photography, and resides in sunny California.

Contact: vhsolutions@yahoo.com
Twitter: @VitalityHealth9